SEX QUIZ FOR COUPLES

Deepening Intimacy and Communication

Bonus:102 sex questions for couples

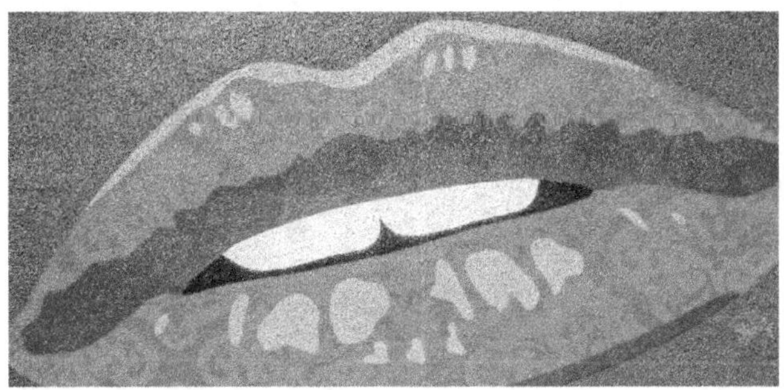

TIM JERRY

TABLE OF CONTENTS

INTRODUCTION

In the realm of human connections, few bonds are as profound and intimate as those shared between couples. The journey of love, trust, and passion intertwines two souls into an inseparable union. At the heart of this beautiful journey lies the delicate art of communication, a key that unlocks the secrets of desire, vulnerability, and pleasure.

Imagine a couple, Alex and Maya, who were once deeply in love but found themselves navigating through the treacherous waters of stagnation. Despite their affection for one another, their once fiery passion seemed to have dimmed, leaving them yearning for a spark that could reignite their intimacy.

One evening, as they were nestled in the warmth of their home, Alex discovered an intriguing book titled Sex Quiz for Couples. The cover exuded an air of mystery and excitement, promising to breathe new life into relationships. Curiosity piqued, Alex shared the discovery with Maya, and they decided to embark on a journey together a journey that would change the course of their relationship forever.

With each question they explored, a world of possibilities unfolded. They found themselves conversing about desires they had never voiced before, confessing hidden fantasies that ignited the embers of passion. The questions probed not only their physical inclinations but also their emotional vulnerabilities, weaving an unbreakable bond between them.

One night, as they delved into a particularly daring question about their secret fantasies, they laughed heartily, realizing they had been sharing similar dreams all along. From that moment, their playful laughter became the soundtrack of their newfound intimacy. The book taught them that vulnerability was not a weakness but a strength—one that allowed them to express their deepest needs without judgment.

As their journey continued, Alex and Maya uncovered the power of emotional intimacy. They learned that being emotionally connected was the gateway to unparalleled physical pleasure, and that understanding each other's love languages could lead to a harmony of desire they had never experienced before.

Through the book's guidance, they overcame challenges that once seemed insurmountable. Open communication enabled them to address issues of mismatched libido and sexual insecurities with compassion and empathy. Instead of viewing obstacles as roadblocks, they began to see them as stepping stones towards a stronger, more resilient bond.

Their shared exploration brought them closer, transforming the act of intimacy into a profound experience of love and mutual respect. The 102 questions were not just conversation starters; they became the threads that intricately woven together the fabric of their relationship.

Intriguingly, the book didn't just focus on physical intimacy but also emphasized the significance of non-sexual touch and affection. Alex and Maya discovered that a simple caress or a gentle hug could speak volumes, nurturing the emotional connection that anchored their love.

As their hearts and bodies intertwined in newfound harmony, they embraced the playfulness of their journey. With a sprinkle of humor and light-heartedness, they discovered that passion thrived in the dance of laughter and joy. Each intimate game they played brought them closer together, reviving the exhilaration of their early days.

Their transformation didn't go unnoticed by their friends and family. Alex and Maya became the epitome of a thriving relationship, inspiring those around them to embark on their own journeys of self-discovery and connection.

As you embark on this remarkable journey, dear reader, with Sex Quiz for Couples as your guide, remember that the power of communication holds the key to unlocking a realm of intimacy you may have never imagined. Open your heart, dare to explore, and let the magic of vulnerability and love guide you on a path of profound and unending connection with your partner. The rewards from the adventure are immeasurable.

CHAPTER 1

Why Communication is Vital in a Relationship

Communication is the lifeblood that courses through the veins of every successful relationship. It is the foundation upon which love, trust, and understanding are built. In the fast-paced world we live in, it's easy to overlook the importance of genuine and open communication between partners. Often, couples may find themselves caught up in their daily routines, leaving little time for meaningful conversations beyond the surface level.

However, when communication falters, the relationship suffers. Unspoken desires, unaddressed concerns, and unresolved conflicts can quietly erode the emotional connection between partners. Without a safe and open space to express themselves, individuals may harbor feelings of loneliness, frustration, or even resentment.

The Art of Active Listening

Effective communication relies heavily on active listening. It goes beyond simply hearing words; it involves being fully present and attentive to what your partner is saying. By practicing active listening, couples can better understand each other's needs and emotions, fostering a deeper level of empathy and support.

Creating a Safe Environment for Honest Dialogue

Building trust is essential in creating a safe environment for honest dialogue. Both partners must feel secure in sharing their thoughts and feelings without fear of judgment or retaliation. Honesty, even when it involves difficult topics, strengthens the bond between couples and allows for authentic growth within the relationship.

The Role of Intimacy in Strengthening Bonds

Intimacy is the soulful connection that binds two individuals together beyond the physical realm. It encompasses emotional, intellectual, and spiritual aspects, weaving an intricate tapestry of shared experiences and understanding. While sexual intimacy is undoubtedly a vital component of romantic relationships, true intimacy extends far beyond the bedroom.

Emotional Intimacy: The Heart-to-Heart Connection

Emotional intimacy involves baring one's innermost thoughts and emotions to a partner without fear of rejection. It requires vulnerability and trust, allowing couples to connect on a profound level. When partners feel emotionally intimate, they can support each other during challenging times and celebrate each other's successes with genuine joy.

Intellectual Intimacy: Stimulating the Mind

Intellectual intimacy thrives on shared interests, stimulating conversations, and a mutual admiration for each other's intellect. Engaging in meaningful discussions, exchanging ideas, and valuing each other's perspectives deepen the connection between partners, fostering an atmosphere of mental stimulation and growth.

As you embark on your journey of exploration and communication, remember that true intimacy flourishes when partners actively listen, communicate openly, and embrace vulnerability. The power of intimate connections lies in their ability to elevate the relationship beyond the ordinary, transforming it into an extraordinary bond that transcends time and trials.

CHAPTER 2

Understanding Each Other's Desires

In the pursuit of a fulfilling and passionate relationship, understanding each other's desires becomes paramount. Beyond the physical realm, desires encompass a wide array of emotional, intellectual, and sensual longings that make each individual unique. Unraveling these desires requires a willingness to communicate openly and without judgment.

Exploring Fantasies and Fetishes

Fantasies and fetishes are aspects of desire that can remain hidden and unspoken, often due to feelings of embarrassment or shame. However, discussing these intimate thoughts with a partner can lead to a newfound sense of trust and intimacy. By sharing fantasies and fetishes, couples may discover common ground, and the act of revealing vulnerability can strengthen their emotional connection.

Discussing Boundaries and Comfort Zones

Within the realm of desires lie boundaries and comfort zones, defining what each partner is willing to explore and what they feel uncomfortable with.

Honest discussions about these limits are essential to maintain respect and trust within the relationship. Understanding and honoring each other's boundaries fosters an environment of safety, enabling partners to express themselves without fear of overstepping limits.

CHAPTER 3

Emotional Connection and Sexuality

The intertwining of emotional connection and sexuality forms the foundation of a deeply satisfying intimate relationship. Beyond the physical act, emotional connection infuses the experience with meaning and depth, elevating sexual encounters to moments of profound intimacy.

How Emotional Intimacy Enhances Sexual Satisfaction

Emotional intimacy cultivates a sense of emotional safety and closeness, which can profoundly impact sexual satisfaction. When partners feel emotionally connected, they are more attuned to each other's needs, desires, and moods. This heightened understanding allows for greater empathy and responsiveness during intimate moments, leading to enhanced pleasure and intimacy.

Sharing Vulnerabilities and Building Trust

Opening up emotionally and sharing vulnerabilities is a powerful way to build trust within a relationship. Vulnerability is an act of courage that allows partners to see each other's authentic selves, free from masks or pretenses. As trust deepens, partners can be more uninhibited and emotionally present during intimate experiences, strengthening the emotional connection that underpins their physical bond.

Understanding each other's desires and fostering emotional connection in a relationship form the core of a truly intimate partnership. Through honest communication and vulnerability, couples can navigate the complexities of desire, boundaries, and emotional closeness, creating a profound and passionate union that stands the test of time.

CHAPTER 4

Communicating Sexual Needs and Preferences

Healthy and fulfilling sexual experiences are nurtured through effective communication of sexual needs and preferences. Openly expressing desires, likes, dislikes, and boundaries with a partner fosters a deeper understanding of each other's wants, leading to a more satisfying intimate connection.

Overcoming Communication Barriers in the Bedroom

Many couples encounter challenges when it comes to discussing their sexual needs within the bedroom. Insecurities, fears of judgment, or societal taboos can create communication barriers. By acknowledging and actively addressing these obstacles, couples can create a safe and non-judgmental space for open dialogue, allowing for the exploration of desires and preferences without hesitation.

Clear and honest communication about likes, dislikes, and wants empowers both partners to cater to each other's pleasure. It paves the way for experimentation and adventure, ensuring that each intimate encounter is tailored to bring maximum satisfaction to both individuals.

CHAPTER 5

Exploring New Territories Together

The path to a dynamic and passionate relationship involves the joint exploration of new territories. Embracing novelty and adventure can breathe fresh excitement into the relationship and reignite the flames of desire.

Trying New Positions and Techniques

Exploring different sexual positions and techniques can add variety and novelty to intimate encounters. By experimenting together, couples can discover new ways to pleasure each other, fostering a sense of excitement and spontaneity in the bedroom.

Incorporating Sensual Games and Toys

Sensual games and toys can infuse playfulness and creativity into the sexual experience. From intimate board games to tasteful adult toys, incorporating these elements can introduce an element of novelty and enhance pleasure, encouraging partners to connect on a deeper level.

CHAPTER 6

Managing Differences in Libido

Sexual desire varies from person to person, and discrepancies in libido can present challenges in a relationship. Addressing these differences with empathy and understanding is crucial to maintaining a harmonious and satisfying sexual connection.

Navigating Mismatches in Sexual Desire

Navigating differences in libido requires open communication and a willingness to compromise. Both partners should feel heard and validated in their feelings, and solutions can be explored together, such as finding middle ground or embracing non-sexual intimacy during times of disparity.

Strategies to Rekindle Passion in the Relationship

Strategies to reignite passion can help couples bridge the gap in libido. This can include creating a romantic atmosphere, prioritizing quality time together, engaging in shared hobbies, or exploring new activities that stimulate emotional and physical intimacy.

CHAPTER 7

Overcoming Sexual Challenges

Sexual challenges are a natural part of many relationships and can stem from various factors, such as physical health, stress, or emotional issues. Tackling these challenges together can strengthen the bond between partners and lead to a deeper understanding of each other's needs.

Addressing Erectile Dysfunction and

Performance Anxiety

Addressing issues like erectile dysfunction and performance anxiety with empathy and support is crucial. Seeking medical advice, counseling, or trying different approaches can assist couples in finding solutions together, reducing pressure and fostering intimacy.

Dealing with Pain or Discomfort During

Intimacy

Pain or discomfort during intimacy can hinder sexual pleasure and emotional connection. Openly discussing these issues with a healthcare professional and a partner can lead to a better understanding of the causes and exploration of alternative approaches to intimacy that prioritize comfort and pleasure.

By openly communicating about sexual needs, exploring new experiences together, and facing challenges as a team, couples can cultivate a thriving and deeply intimate relationship that stands the test of time.

CHAPTER 8

Intimacy Beyond the Physical

While physical intimacy is an essential aspect of any romantic relationship, it is equally important to recognize that intimacy extends far beyond the physical realm. True intimacy encompasses emotional connection, trust, and a sense of security, making it the foundation for a deeply fulfilling and lasting partnership.

The Importance of Non-Sexual Touch and Affection

Non-sexual touch and affection are powerful expressions of love and care. Holding hands, hugging, cuddling, and even a gentle touch on the arm can communicate emotions that words often fail to convey. These acts of physical tenderness nurture emotional bonds, fostering a deeper connection between partners.

Cultivating Intimacy Through Emotional Connection

Emotional connection is the heart of intimacy. It involves sharing one's innermost thoughts, fears, dreams, and vulnerabilities with a partner, knowing that they will be met with love and understanding. By cultivating emotional intimacy, couples build a solid foundation for trust and support, allowing them to navigate life's challenges together with greater resilience.

Understanding that intimacy goes beyond mere physical contact empowers couples to prioritize emotional connection and non-sexual touch. Embracing these aspects of intimacy leads to a more profound and meaningful bond, enriching both partners' lives and creating a relationship filled with love, trust, and lasting happiness.

CHAPTER 9

Deepening Intimacy with Communication Exercises

Effective communication is the key to unlocking a deeper level of intimacy in any relationship. Communication exercises provide a structured and intentional way for couples to explore their feelings, desires, and aspirations, fostering a stronger emotional connection and a greater understanding of each other.

The 36 Questions to Fall in Love

The 36 Questions to Fall in Love is a renowned psychological study that offers a series of progressively intimate questions designed to accelerate emotional closeness between two people. By engaging in these thought-provoking and personal questions, couples can delve into each other's thoughts and emotions, creating a shared vulnerability that strengthens their emotional bond.

Mindful Listening and Empathetic Responding

Mindful listening and empathetic responding are invaluable communication tools that enhance intimacy. Being fully present during conversations, giving undivided attention, and showing genuine empathy when responding to a partner's emotions can create a safe space for open and honest dialogue. These practices nurture trust and emotional connection, promoting a deeper understanding of each other's needs and desires.

By actively engaging in communication exercises and practicing mindful listening, couples can transcend superficial conversations and embark on a journey of profound emotional intimacy. These exercises offer an opportunity to connect on a deeper level, bringing partners closer together and solidifying the foundation of their relationship.

CONCLUSION

The journey of exploring sex quiz for couples is an expedition into the heart of intimacy and communication. It is a testament to the beauty and complexity of human connections, as partners navigate the intricacies of desire, vulnerability, and love.

Embracing Growth and Change in Your Sexual Journey

Any healthy partnership must embrace development and change. As individuals and couples evolve over time, so too will their desires, needs, and preferences. Being open to this evolution creates a space for continual growth, exploration, and deeper intimacy.

The Ongoing Adventure of Intimacy and Love

Intimacy and love are an ongoing adventure, one that transcends the boundaries of time. Nurturing the emotional and physical bond between partners requires constant effort, dedication, and a commitment to understanding and supporting each other's journey.

In the pursuit of a fulfilling and passionate relationship, remember that effective communication, emotional connection, and a willingness to explore and adapt are the cornerstones of intimacy. By embracing vulnerability, sharing desires, and appreciating each other's unique qualities, couples can forge a love that not only withstands the test of time but also thrives in its depth and richness. As you embark on your own journey of discovery and connection, may you find joy, growth, and boundless love with your partner.

1. What are your preferred methods of expressing love?

2. How do you feel loved and appreciated?

3. What physical touch makes you feel most connected?

4. What are your sexual desires and fantasies?

5. How can we create a safe space to discuss our intimate needs?

6. How often would you like to have intimate moments?

7. How do you feel about initiating intimacy?

8. Do you prefer verbal or non-verbal cues to express intimacy?

9. How can we explore new experiences in the bedroom?

10. What are your thoughts on setting boundaries in the bedroom?

11. What do you think about shows of affection in public?

12. What are your views on sharing sexual fantasies with each other?

13. How do you want to address any sexual concerns or issues that arise?

14. What do you find most attractive about each other?

15. How can we maintain intimacy during stressful times?

16. What are your preferred methods of sexual communication?

17. How can we maintain intimacy as we age?

18. What are your thoughts on trying new positions or techniques?

19. How do you feel about using sex toys in the bedroom?

20. How can we ensure that both partners feel satisfied and fulfilled?

21. How do you define emotional intimacy in the context of our relationship?

22. What are your views on masturbation within a relationship?

23. How can we ensure open and honest communication about our desires?

24. What can we do to make each other feel more desirable?

25. How do you feel about scheduling intimate moments in our busy lives?

26. What are your views on pornography within a relationship?

27. How can we support each other's sexual boundaries and limits?

28. What can we do to maintain passion and excitement in our relationship?

29. How do you feel about cuddling and physical affection outside of intimacy?

30. How can we be more adventurous in our sexual relationship?

31. What are your thoughts on practicing mindfulness during intimate moments?

32. How can we incorporate more romance into our relationship?

33. What are your favorite ways to initiate intimacy?

34. How do you feel about sending flirtatious or suggestive messages to each other?

35. How can we create a more romantic atmosphere in the bedroom?

36. What are your views on engaging in role-play or sexual fantasies together?

37.How do you feel about trying new experiences, such as bondage or blindfolding?

38.What are your thoughts on introducing massage or sensual touch into our relationship?

39. How can we maintain a healthy balance between intimacy and other aspects of our relationship?

40. What are your views on engaging in sexual acts outside of intercourse?

41. How do you feel about engaging in mutual self-pleasure together?

42. What are your thoughts on cuddling and non-sexual physical affection?

43. How can we express gratitude for each other in the context of intimacy?

44. What are your views on engaging in spontaneous intimate moments?

45. How do you feel about sharing sexual fantasies that involve other people?

46. How can we support each other's emotional needs in the bedroom?

47. What are your thoughts on taking breaks from intimacy if one partner needs it?

48. How do you feel about incorporating aphrodisiacs or mood enhancers into our intimate moments?

49. How can we prioritize self-care to improve our intimate relationship?

50. What are your views on engaging in intimate activities while on vacation or in new environments?

51. What are your thoughts on initiating intimacy through surprise gestures or notes?

52. How can we incorporate more laughter and playfulness into our intimate moments?

53. What are your views on watching romantic movies or reading erotic literature together?

54. How do you feel about engaging in intimate activities in the great outdoors?

55. How can we express love and appreciation for each other outside of the bedroom?

56. What are your thoughts on taking turns planning intimate date nights or getaways?

57. How do you feel about engaging in physical activities together to increase intimacy?

58. How can we create a relaxing and comfortable space for intimate moments?

59. What are your views on maintaining intimacy during times of physical separation?

60. How do you feel about exploring tantric practices or deepening our connection spiritually?

61. What are your thoughts on setting goals for improving intimacy in our relationship?

62. How can we prioritize self-awareness and personal growth within our intimate relationship?

63. What are your views on seeking professional help, such as therapy, to enhance intimacy?

64. How do you feel about engaging in intimate moments after an argument or disagreement?

65. How can we express gratitude for each other's efforts in the context of intimacy?

66. What are your thoughts on maintaining intimacy after having children?

67. How do you feel about creating a shared intimate space, such as a designated "love nest"?

68. What are your views on engaging in intimate activities while on a retreat or spiritual journey?

69. How can we ensure that we both feel secure and confident in our intimate moments?

70. What are your thoughts on taking turns fulfilling each other's desires and fantasies?

71. How do you feel about engaging in intimate moments as a form of stress relief?

72. How can we communicate our boundaries and comfort levels during intimate activities?

73. How can we incorporate music or sensual playlists into our intimate moments?

74. What are your views on engaging in intimate activities as a way to express forgiveness and healing?

75. How do you feel about exploring different types of touch and affection during intimacy?

76. How can we surprise each other with gestures of appreciation and love in the bedroom?

77. What are your thoughts on experimenting with different scents and aromatherapy to enhance intimacy?

78. How do you feel about engaging in intimate moments after a long day at work or a tiring event?

79. How can we create a more intimate and personal connection through deep conversations?

80. What are your views on taking turns planning surprise date nights to keep the spark alive?

81. How do you feel about engaging in intimate activities that involve laughter and humor?

82. How can we celebrate special occasions in a way that strengthens our intimate bond?

83. What are your thoughts on engaging in intimate moments that involve exploration and curiosity?

84. How do you feel about incorporating elements of role reversal or power dynamics in our intimate relationship?

85. How can we communicate our love and affection through gestures and actions, both inside and outside the bedroom?

86. What are your views on using intimate moments as an opportunity for personal growth and vulnerability?

87. How do you feel about exploring new erogenous zones and sensitive areas on each other's bodies?

88. How can we maintain a sense of spontaneity and excitement in our intimate relationship?

89. What are your thoughts on engaging in intimate moments that promote relaxation and stress relief?

90. How do you feel about incorporating elements of fantasy and imagination into our intimate activities?

91. How can we express our desires and boundaries in a way that fosters mutual understanding and respect?

92. What are your views on engaging in intimate activities that involve light bondage or sensory play?

93. How do you feel about taking turns planning surprise getaways or romantic weekends together?

94. How can we create a deeper emotional connection through our intimate moments?

95. What are your thoughts on expressing appreciation and admiration for each other's physical appearance?

96 How do you feel about engaging in intimate moments as a means of celebration and joy?

97. How can we communicate our sexual needs and preferences in a non-judgmental and open manner?

98. What are your views on using intimate moments as a form of stress relief and emotional release?

99. How do you feel about exploring different forms of touch, such as gentle and sensual touch or more passionate and intense touch?

100. How can we incorporate more appreciation and gratitude for each other's efforts in our intimate relationship?

101. What are your views on engaging in intimate moments that involve creative and artistic expressions of love?

102. How do you feel about exploring different forms of physical affection and touch outside of the bedroom to strengthen our emotional bond?